Living Positively

Ayelah Iqbal

ISBN:153749418X
ISBN-13:9781537494180

DEDICATION

I'd like to dedicate this to my mother- who has always encouraged me to live a positive and happy life.

CONTENTS

PREFACE

Most people have the common misconception that positivity is innate; they believe that some people are born positive while others are not. I can say for a fact that I was not born positive. I spent my middle school years with a negative attitude that tainted many aspects of my life. It was as if I wasn't allowing myself to be happy. I had yet to learn the importance of appreciation and positive thinking that transform a mundane life into a happy one. At the end of the day, chances are that the happiest person on Earth lives a similar life to your own. The difference between being happy and unhappy depends on how you view yourself and your situation. Through years of research and reading, I learned that I needed an attitude transformation. The transformation didn't happen all at once, but I slowly began to change my attitude through practice and began to incorporate small measures in my life to make me happier. I can say with certainty that I am not the same girl that I was a few years ago- I am infinitely more self confident and happy. I am optimistic about my current situation and my future and am excited to learn more and experience new endeavors. I owe this change and excitement to the science behind positive thinking.

BECOMING WHO YOU WANT TO BE

"If you don't like something, change it. If you can't, change your attitude." —Maya Angelou

I know, we've all heard this one a million times. But this quote hits home with me because without knowing it, I've been living it for the past few years. It all started when I started to reinvent myself. Now I don't mean completely transforming myself like movie characters do. I mean that I put aside my insecurities and allowed myself to become the person that I had always wanted to be. I changed the aspects of myself that I wasn't happy with, and if I couldn't change something, I changed my attitude toward it.

People often say you should accept who you are, and not change anything. While I agree that it's important to accept yourself, it's also true that sometimes if you change something about yourself, you can love yourself even more. At the end of the day, every one of us will find fault in ourselves, it's human nature—and if we can change these faults while remaining healthy, then I think we owe it to ourselves to be the best that we can be. Keep in mind that I'm emphasizing that we should remain healthy, both physically and emotionally. If at any point you are endangering your health, you are essentially trying to change something that you can't change.

For me, I started off by letting my true personality show. I had always been quiet, and saw myself as an introvert. I acted subdued and kept my thoughts to myself, which went against my true nature and who I wanted to be. I didn't have a sudden realization that I needed to embody my true extroverted nature—instead I slowly started to realize that I didn't want to be the person that I was acting like. Hiding behind shyness was just a safety net that allowed me to not put myself out there, and while it was safe, it wasn't making me happy. So, I started to break out of my shell, and although it was different, it was nice to finally be myself. It's refreshing to be the person that you want to be after hiding for so long.

However, I can't take all the credit for my transformation—I also have to thank my support system. I put myself in an environment that allowed for growth, and surrounded myself with people that brought out the best in me. (Thank you, friends!) They pushed me to become a better person, and they brought out my true personality without even knowing it. As trite as this sounds, I didn't have to try to be myself around them—I just was myself. I decided to be the person that I wanted to be, and I surrounded myself with people that facilitated this process. I wasn't happy with myself, so I decided to change. I wasn't happy with the effects that my environment had on me, so I changed my environment.

I understand that we may not all be able to change our environment, but that's where the second half of the quote comes in: changing your attitude. Obviously there were some parts of my environment that I couldn't change (for example, I couldn't change the fact that many people still saw me as an introvert because of my past actions), but I had to change my attitude about it. Instead of trying to change how everyone saw me, I focused on letting my true personality show and accepted the fact that I couldn't control people's thoughts about me. Some people would realize that I was actually an extrovert, while others would assume that I was shy and quiet, but it didn't matter because I couldn't change it. At the end of the day, my opinion of myself was infinitely more important than other people's opinions of me.

The second part of my transformation was a physical one. We all have physical insecurities that inhibit us from being as confident as we can be; we wouldn't be human without them. Some of these insecurities can be changed, while others are indelible and are just a part of who we are. The key is to change what you can, and accept what you can't. I started off by trying to change my skin. I had struggled with acne for years and it had taken its toll on my self-esteem. That year, I decided to visit a dermatologist and fix the root of my problem.

Clearing my skin was not a quick fix. The dermatologist prescribed numerous gels and antibiotics; some worked and some didn't. I even experienced an allergic reaction to one of the antibiotics (my face swelled up like a red balloon, it wasn't pretty). But eventually, a precarious balance of gels and antibiotics yielded results and I now have fairly clear skin. My "transformation" wasn't complete, but this success motivated me to make other changes.

I haven't been able to change all my insecurities—take my hair, for example. Naturally, I have thick, wavy hair. I've wished for straight hair all my life. I've tried everything to get straight hair—keratin treatments, products, heatless techniques—and none of it worked. I even went through a period of time when I straightened my hair almost every day. Finally, I decided to accept it. Easier said than done. It was a slow process, which began with wearing my hair natural. At first I hated it, but eventually I began to see the beauty of my natural hair, and people around me saw it too. This may sound vain, but I really do have pretty hair. It curls in loose waves that look like they've been heat-styled, and they aren't even frizzy. Although it took a while for me to see this, now I cherish my natural hair and wouldn't trade it for anything else. It's funny how things work out when you force them to.

Allowing myself to become who I want to be has made me feel like I am truly the person that I was born to be. As cliché as it sounds, at the end of the day it's your opinion of yourself that matters the most, and I have a great opinion of myself now that I believe I embody the person that I really am. This process has taken time and energy, but I believe that it has made me happier in the long run. It has also helped me discover parts of myself that I didn't know existed—I don't think I would have started writing if I didn't let my true personality show. If you feel as if you haven't been the person that you truly are, I encourage you to change it, to be the person that you want to be.

PURSUING A PASSION

The word "passion" has become so cliché. For example, how many times have I heard someone say something like, "I'm so passionate about soccer." In my mind, that could mean a variety of things. It could mean that the person enjoys playing soccer, is good at playing soccer, enjoys following soccer, or is *actually passionate* about soccer. The dictionary describes "passion" as the object of a strong fondness or desire, but I characterize it differently: something that evokes an intense urge to engage in anything related to it. Being passionate about soccer, for example, might mean that you would like to play soccer, watch soccer, learn about soccer players, and follow soccer tournaments. (Maybe not *all* of those things, but definitely some of them.)

Most of us aren't born with passions. Unless you're training to be an Olympic medalist or you've invented something, chances are you're just like the rest of us, drifting from one interest to another without a clear devotion to a single activity. That's totally normal and okay. We can't expect ourselves to develop passions. Instead, all we can do is feed our likes in hopes that they will germinate into loves. If you enjoy watching TV, try writing a screenplay. If you love fashion, create a website documenting your outfits. You can pursue multiple interests until you find one that resonates with you; pursuing an interest provides a similar happiness boost that pursuing a passion does, and it teaches you invaluable information about yourself along the way.

We all know that we derive pleasure from doing activities that we enjoy. Now double that amount of pleasure. That's approximately the amount of pleasure that we get from pursuing something that we are passionate about. However, occasionally indulging in a passion and actively pursuing it are completely different things. In order to fully pursue a passion, you need to treat it like a priority, and give it as much effort and time as you would any other responsibility. I know, very few of us have large amounts of free time on our hands, but I encourage you to find time to further your personal curiosity. You might have to cut down on other activities, but I promise that the fulfillment you'll get from your passion will be unmatched.

Committing to a big project can provide a sense of structure to pursuing your passion and ensure that you take part in it frequently. In my case, I combined a love for psychology and writing by tackling a large project: writing a collection of essays. If I wasn't writing these essays, I probably wouldn't find the time to read books about happiness or work on improving my writing skills. Sometimes, all you need is something big and exciting to guide you in the right direction. In addition, tackling a large project and completing it provides a happiness boost in itself, from achieving a goal. As soon as I complete an essay, a flood of calming and fulfilling emotions washes over me; sometimes the anticipation of this feeling is enough to keep me writing despite a hectic schedule. These essays have given me a sense of purpose that boosts my happiness every day. Whatever your passion may be—whether it's following sports, running, or even gardening—making it a central part of your life will have long-lasting effects on your happiness.

I encourage you to experiment with interests until you find a passion. It may take some time, but it's worth it, because it will provide you with constant satisfaction and ensure that you don't get stuck in a routine that bores you. Once you find it, even one free hour to explore it can be thrilling. After all, life is about finding and acting on what you love.

BEING AWARE

The dictionary defines being aware as having knowledge, being conscious, or being cognizant. While all three of these definitions are true, awareness is not just a state of being but a way of thinking that affects every moment of your life. When you are mentally aware, your senses are all tuned in to every variation and detail in the environment around you. You experience every single emotion that arises within you and every single stimulus that appears in the environment. It's as if you are one with your surroundings and have a perfect understanding of yourself.

While it might not seem like being aware has anything to do with being happy, it is in fact essential, because unaware people don't feel as happy as aware people do. Aware people allow emotions to consume them, while most people skim over or suppress their feelings because it's easier. Truly feeling your emotions allows you to fully experience them and be in tune with what causes them. If you know exactly what causes your happiness, you can more easily create these conditions again. Of course, truly feeling your emotions means not only that when you're happy, you're on top of the world, but also that when you're sad you feel every painful sting. Yes, this is more painful and more difficult, but another way of looking at it is that the contrast between sadness and happiness makes us appreciate happiness even more. Think of it this way: if your emotions never changed, there would be no happiness. And anyway, while I agree that sadness can be difficult, it's also a part of life—you aren't truly living unless you feel it.

This is definitely easier said than done, but I am proud to say that I've tried to incorporate it into my life as much as I can. I became aware by fully immersing myself into every situation and every emotion. This isn't a physical change as much as a mental one. Whereas sometimes I used to be tuned out mentally, I now physically experience every moment of my life. I force myself to think about every situation that I'm in and every emotion that I'm feeling. Yes, it is difficult and more painful, but I have learned a lot more about myself through this process. I've learned what kind of situations make me happy and sad, and this has affected my journey in life. I now know that I am content when I'm exploring new places, so I surround myself with people who are ready to explore with me. I've also learned that I become sad when I don't experience a change of pace, so I make sure that every few days I experience something new. My goal is not to eradicate sadness, but to encourage happiness and truly feel both emotions when they arise.

Being aware can also increase your understanding of the world around you. If you are fully aware of all the nuances of a situation, you understand the situation infinitely more than someone who just skims over it. This applies to everything from understanding how to excel in your given position to knowing how to navigate a particular situation.

Being aware even allowed me to secure a prestigious internship over applicants that were more qualified than I. My awareness allowed me to pick up on subtle indicators throughout my interview that showed me what kind of intern the company was looking for. For example, I noticed that the interviewer kept asking me questions about how I would approach different situations or problems, which made me realize that the company wanted someone who approached a situation multiple ways to find the optimum solution. This allowed me to highlight my creativity, positive attitude, and determination in ways that many other applicants probably didn't. Although I was probably not totally qualified for the position, my awareness throughout the interview allowed me to impress the interviewer. I wouldn't have noticed the subtle details in the interviewer's queries if I hadn't been fully immersed in the situation.

Being aware has also allowed me to understand particular situations infinitely more than I would have if I were unaware. For example, I recently analyzed a friend's behavior to fully understand her state of mind. It was prom season and every girl was talking and thinking about who she wanted to be asked by. My friend and I approached another friend, let's call her Jane, and asked Jane who she wanted to ask her to prom. Of course, my friend and I already had a sneaking suspicion that Jane wanted to be asked by a specific boy, but we said nothing. Jane insisted that she didn't want to be asked by anyone, so it would be less awkward for her to go alone. My friend and I were puzzled, so we began to analyze her actions. Our observations were contrary to everything that she had said. We watched her flirt with the same boy every single day and even heard her joke about being his girlfriend. That was proof enough for us. We didn't want to meddle in our friend's life, but at the same time we were certain of what she wanted because we tuned ourselves in to every situation. We began to subtly hint to the boy that he should ask Jane to prom and come in our group, and he decided to, admitting that he wouldn't have thought to ask Jane if we hadn't suggested it. She later admitted to us that she lied because she didn't think that this boy would ask her. Because we were fully aware, we noticed details and nuances in her behavior, and acting on these details completely changed Jane's prom experience and genuinely made her happy.

Being aware has an infinite amount of positive consequences, many of which I haven't even experienced yet, but it begins with immersing yourself in the present. Deeply thinking about every emotion that you feel allows you to understand yourself on a deep level, and to fully experience every emotion that life has to offer and get the most out of every experience. Being aware allows you to understand people and the world around you more deeply too. The world has an endless amount of possibilities, and we have access to more of them when we fully immerse ourselves in all that life has to offer.

CURIOSITY

Ever since I was in middle school, my father has been telling me to be curious and to pursue the things I'm curious about. At first, I had no clue what he meant. I understood what being curious meant, I just had no idea how to apply it to my life or why it was important to. I knew that curiosity was innate, so it seemed almost unnecessary to focus my attention on it. And so, being the immature girl that I was, I nodded my head in agreement every time my father mentioned curiosity even though I had no clue what he meant.

I finally truly experienced curiosity when I stumbled upon it on my own. One summer, something struck me in an article about technology on Engadget (my favorite website at the time). One article led to several articles and soon I was writing my own articles and reaching out to technology bloggers. The best part is, I wasn't even conscious that this was a sign of curiosity at the time—I was just doing what felt right. Now, looking back, I realize that I've had this curiosity in me for a long time, it's just been dormant for the past couple of years.

I have to admit, in high school I got so caught up with my grades and social standing that I stopped making time for things that genuinely sparked my interest. Looking back, I can't remember ever being less happy than I was at this time. My priorities were clouded and I genuinely felt as if I wasn't *really living*. I was living life, but I wasn't experiencing it the way it was meant to be experienced. The upside is that this unhappiness is what reminded me of the importance of curiosity and spurred me to start reading about it. I realized that I wasn't the only one who felt stifled by the lack of curiosity in my life— many other people were longing for the same sense of freedom and adventure. Curiosity is a liberating element that opens you up to a world of new opportunities, and I was wasting my life by shutting myself down to it. That's when I decided to start pursuing anything and everything that sparked my interest.

But curiosity doesn't end there. It isn't about finding something you like and then focusing all your attention on it while shutting out other possibilities—it's about constantly being open to new opportunities. That's the beauty of curiosity: *It never ends.* It hinges on the fact that your journey isn't over, and never will be over, which forces you to constantly try to find a new path. Curiosity is about questioning known facts just for the hell of it, just in case you learn something new or find another way of looking at something. It's about experimenting and constantly finding events and opportunities that make you happy. You can't plan for curiosity, so you might as well enjoy the ride. I think that's my favorite thing about it: there is no possible way to set a goal because you don't know what kinds of things you are going to encounter. I could never have predicted that reading a book about happiness would inspire me to write my own, and I can't predict what kinds of opportunities will come knocking on my door after I write this book. The beauty of opening myself up to new things is that I don't know what effects these opportunities will have on my future. But I definitely do know that these opportunities wouldn't have arisen if I hadn't opened myself up to curiosity.

Now that we've talked about the wonders of curiosity, you're probably wondering how to integrate it into your mentality. Personally, I started off by reminding myself to see each new experience as an opportunity to exercise curiosity. If I enjoyed an article about astronomy, I would read another and see if it piqued my interest. If I was taking my dog for a walk, I would take a different turn into a field and see where it took me. (I now love taking my dog for a walk in that field and found a nearby forest alongside a river—it's so beautiful that it's surreal.) Granted, being curious was a bit more time consuming and harder than sticking with my everyday routine, but it was infinitely more fulfilling than walking my dog on the same trail every single day.

I also believe that becoming curious means constantly questioning things and asking yourself what comes next. If you open yourself up to new endeavors and possibilities by actively searching for them, then you're infinitely more likely to find them. But don't confuse thinking about the future with not being satisfied in the present. The question shouldn't be, "How can I improve my situation?" but instead "How can I grow?" The difference between these two questions is that the second shows appreciation for the present while the first signals an urgency to make things better. It's a subtle difference, but an appreciation for the present is extremely important when it comes to being happy.

Curiosity is now here to stay in my life. It opens up a world of possibilities and allows people to truly grow in ways they could never have imagined. It also helps you think about the world in a different, more positive way. I can attest to the fact that curiosity has made me a happier and more content person. I appreciate every second of the present and am also excited to see what kind of opportunities the future has to offer. There are now things on my radar that I never would have even considered in the past. Curiosity is truly fulfilling, and now I see what my dad had been talking about for all those years..

CHARITY

The idea that "charity" can make you feel happier has been around since the beginning of time. It's a fundamental in many religions; Christianity preaches that people should give in order to attain eternal salvation. Kids are taught to share from birth, and this idea is fostered into adulthood, when adults are encouraged to give to the less fortunate. But charity benefits both parties, the giver and the receiver. If you can do something that benefits yourself and others, then I think you've found the perfect balance.

One of the main kinds of emotional "charity" can be defined by the Confucian teaching of *ren,* or benevolence. This teaching stresses the importance of treating people with compassion, which I believe is one of the most important ways to spread positivity and happiness, and being a force of good in other people's lives. Personally, I believe this to be extremely fulfilling and equally as beneficial as monetary assistance. Emotional benevolence is something we can all provide, and it's deeply needed in this world. How many times have you noticed someone that obviously craves advice or just needs a confidante? Even with seven billion people on the planet, there seems to be a shortage of sympathetic ears.

So, if you see an opportunity to be a force of good in someone's life, I urge you to give it a try. Being there for someone not only makes them feel happier, it also makes you feel more fulfilled yourself. Just yesterday, I received a text from a friend asking if I could give her friend some advice. Although I didn't know this other girl and had no reason to help her, I agreed to lending her some of my time on a whim. The three of us talked on the phone for an hour about her "boy troubles" and eventually came to a conclusion. I didn't know this girl at all previous to our conversation, but we shared some laughs and I gained a new friend from the experience. After the phone call, she was content that she had gained a new friend and some advice, and I was happy that I got to know her and managed to help her. This kind of happiness is underrated, but I have to say that it's one of the purest forms. Any situation that benefits both parties immensely and spreads positivity is a good idea in my book.

In Buddhism, one of the main forms of *dana,* or charity, is monetary assistance. Even today, monetary assistance can be a solution to some of the most prevalent problems in our society, whether it be world hunger or a lack of vaccinations available for children. On a smaller scale, there are people in all of our communities that could use a helping hand. Most religions, including Buddhism, teach followers that they should give a portion of their earnings to these causes, whether it be to attain salvation or happiness. However, even many religious people tend to forget this fundamental teaching as they get caught up in their daily lives. Although I'm not particularly religious, I have been trying to make a concerted effort to be more monetarily generous, not just with causes but also with people that I know. Whenever I donate to charity, I feel content because I believe that I'm doing the right thing and fulfilling my duty as a good world citizen. I also take pleasure in knowing that I am doing my part to alleviate a problem that plagues many. However, when I spend money on people that I'm close to, I feel a different kind of happiness. This happiness isn't derived from a sense of duty, but rather just pure happiness at seeing someone that I love smile. One of my most vivid memories is when I bought my brother his birthday gift last year. I bought him a set of expensive speakers that he had been wanting for months but hadn't had the money to buy for himself. Since I had a summer job, I decided to spend some of my money to get him a meaningful gift. When he opened the gift, I saw a pure smile on his face that instantly filled me with happiness and made every cent I spent worth it.

There are many ways to be a force of good in other people's lives, so I urge you to experiment until you find something that works for you. I can say from personal experience that helping people has a way of making you feel a pure form of happiness that you never get sick of. But the best part is, you are not only deriving happiness but also giving it to others.

THE LITTLE THINGS

We live each day waiting for the big moments, whether it's Friday night plans, a vacation, or even just waiting to get home and sleep. Sure, it gives us something to look forward to, but this anticipation causes us to overlook the small moments that make up our everyday lives. Big moments make up only a small fraction of our lives, and by concentrating on them we let daily joys slip through our fingertips.

I have definitely been a victim of this way of thinking. Take prom, for example. My friends and I spent months waiting for prom. So many times we said, "We just need to get through these next couple of weeks, then we'll have prom." Those weeks were painful and slow—but only because we dreaded every minute of them. Sure, we were stressed about tests, sleep-deprived, and sick of prom planning, but that doesn't excuse the fact that we truly had awful attitudes towards those few weeks ahead—weeks that made up significantly more time than prom ever did. The ironic part is, prom did not live up to our expectations—in fact, it was pretty boring.

Our lives are made up of small, seemingly insignificant moments, with big events sporadically peppered in between. Next time you and your friends are aimlessly talking in the hallway, take some time to actually enjoy their company, and immerse yourself in the conversation, even if it is aimless banter. Our attitude toward the more-mundane events of our lives is what determines whether we appreciate them or not. Dreading or ignoring the small moments deprives us of the positivity and laughter that they offer us; we should be absorbing all the positivity that we can.

Our society tends to prioritize the big, memorable moments in life. You rarely hear people talk about how great a run made them feel, or how nice it was to sit and talk with a friend for 10 minutes. Instead we talk about how amazing a party was or how much we got to relax on vacation. We are expected, in this society, to spend our present planning for our future. Instead, I think we have to find a balance between planning for the future and enjoying the present.

Personally, I've had a busy year and will continue to. My classmates and I are at a crucial stage in our lives, where we're preparing for and applying to colleges. But I've realized that although I do need to consider my future, and am anxiously awaiting acceptance (or rejection) letters, I also need to focus on enjoying the present. My life for the next year may lead up to a college decision, but it will be made up of small moments that I vow to value. I truly believe that this perspective will help me remain happy even in times of stress.

Life is essentially a collection of moments. By disregarding small moments, we are disregarding life. So next time you are sitting in class, waiting to go home, try to shift your attitude and enjoy the people sitting next to you and the environment around you. This could be one of the moments that adds joy to your everyday life and makes you a happier person.

EXPRESSING GRATITUDE TO OTHERS

Sometimes our lives get so busy and we get so stuck in our routines, it's easy to forget to appreciate the light that people bring to our lives. Life is just a series of events, peppered with moments of joy and love. Even though we might feel immense pleasure while talking to a close friend, we can take it for granted, and the moment becomes just another in the midst of a busy day. Forgotten moments like these are the ones that truly give us happiness. The transient nature of these moments should motivate us to appreciate the positivity that we enjoy and the people that bring it to our lives. That's why I believe in savoring every one of these moments and realizing just how much joy interaction with loved ones can give you.

Appreciating these moments and appreciating the people that make up these moments are two completely different things. It's important to express gratitude not only for the moment, but for the person that helps create the moment—because they are bringing us joy. It's easy to forget the loved ones that bring light to our lives and I think that we owe it to them to express gratitude once in a while. I can't tell you how many times I've thoroughly enjoyed spending time with someone, but not told them. Now, looking back, I feel like I cheated them out of knowing how much they mean to me. I know it might feel weird to thank people for their company, but I promise that this small expression of gratitude can do wonders for your attitude and theirs. It puts life in perspective and helps you enjoy the moment, and it makes the other person feel happy and appreciated. Recently, I've been trying to make a concerted effort to show appreciation for my friends and family. It's definitely outside social convention, but I think it's been beneficial for me to express my real thoughts and feelings to the people that I care about.

Although I have been trying to incorporate this gratitude into my routine for a while, I didn't truly realize just how important it was until someone expressed gratitude to me. My friend and I were getting ice cream after not having spent time with each other in a while. We had spent an hour talking about mundane stuff, which led to hysterically laughing with tears in our eyes. It was one of those moments where you just feel blissfully happy and content. Right before we were about to say good-bye, she told me that she was happy that we had spent some time together and that she was thankful to have me as a close friend. That single sentence immediately put a smile on my face. I felt appreciated and thankful for our friendship, and even closer to my friend. It's amazing how one second of openness and pure honesty brings two people together. Maybe it seems like a sudden expression of gratitude might feel awkward, but the fact that it was just so honest and so kind prevented it from being weird—just the opposite, it brought us closer together. Sometimes sharing your innermost thoughts and showing some vulnerability can take you to a deeper and more fulfilling place.

That was the moment when I truly realized how important it was to tell people how much they meant to me. Prior to this conversation, I had just been experimenting with gratitude and hadn't truly realized its importance and impact. This moment showed me that I needed to express gratitude for these small moments of happiness and for the people that bring them into my life. It was an awakening moment, because it's changed my outlook. At the end of the day, openness and vulnerability bring not only us, but other people happiness. In my case, it not only made my day but also strengthened a friendship.

TACKLING A PROJECT

Motivation can be hard to come by. Often, by the time you've completed your responsibilities there's not much energy left to tackle anything else, especially a large project. While I do believe that it's important to take time out to rest, I also think it's essential to stay productive.

Personally, if I take too much time off, I start to feel sluggish and bored. Last summer I decided to take a month off to rejuvenate and relax. I spent the entire four weeks watching TV, going out to eat with friends, and sleeping. At the end of the first week I felt relaxed and content. A week later, I was starting to feel bored and sluggish. At the end of the third week, I was desperate to do something even slightly productive.

The solution for my sluggishness was a workout schedule. Obviously working out is known to counteract laziness, but I attribute the alleviation of my boredom to the simple fact that I was doing something productive. The fact that I was leaving the house every day to pursue something beneficial gave me a sense of satisfaction that was infinitely more comforting than spending another day at home watching TV. I was happy knowing that I was spending my time wisely, and this small dose of productivity inspired me to pursue other tasks or projects (whereas lazing around at home only made me feel more sluggish). I began to read books about topics that interested me, which led me to books about the psychology of happiness. That's when I got the idea to write these essays!

According to Brett Blumenthal, people feel happy through the pursuit of accomplishments and fulfilling goals. Setting goals provides a sense of structure that helps you accomplish them more easily, which in turn provides a surge of confidence. I think we can all attest to the fact that we feel proud and happy when we accomplish something that's important to us. Personally, ever since I was a young kid goals have motivated me. Whether it was getting an A on a particular assignment or scoring a goal in a soccer match, there's always been something tangible that I've been working toward. There's something about being able to see the metaphorical light at the end of the tunnel that motivates people to actually get there. And when we get there, knowing that our dedication and hard work has earned us something tangible is one of the purest forms of happiness. An obvious example is the college admissions process. I watched a friend work tirelessly for years and years toward her goal of getting into her dream school, despite crippling stress and exhaustion. The hard work was painful, but once she got her acceptance letter she was euphoric. I've never seen someone so happy.

Whether it's getting into your dream school or going for a run every day, I urge you to consider pursuing a goal. It may seem like spending that time doing nothing might make you happier, but trust me when I say that doing nothing gets old quickly. It's infinitely more satisfying to work toward a goal that can you make you feel proud of yourself.

DAILY REFLECTIONS

Sometimes we get so caught up in our everyday routines that we forget to take a step back and reflect on what we're thankful for. Gratitude for and awareness of the positive aspects of your life instantly changes your attitude, and allows you to fully feel the happiness in your life. There is positivity to be found in every day and every experience—at least a lesson to be learned or something to be gained, no matter how small. No matter how bad your day feels, it will always help to forget the negative for a little while and focus on the big picture. Even in my times of hopelessness, reflecting on the positives in my life can bring me joy.

There are many ways to reflect on what you are thankful for. Some people choose to spend a few minutes a day to reflect on the day's positives, while others choose to spend hours in meditation or prayer. Many of us don't have hours to spend, so a small chunk of time will do. Personally, I like to write down a short list of things I'm thankful for, at least once or twice a week. I've found this to be deeply fulfilling. It helps me focus on the positives in my life and highlights my personal growth in a meaningful way. Nowadays, there are plenty of apps that you can use to write these reflections in, but a plain notebook works just as well. Both allow you to make personal reflection a habit and to read previous entries to see how far you've come.

Even if you don't choose to write down what you're thankful for, thinking about it is also beneficial. Mental reflection gets you into the habit of showing appreciation for things as they occur. I can't tell you how many times I've been in a situation and, in the moment, realized that I'm truly grateful for the experience. This shift in awareness hasn't been easy—it's taken a lot of practice, believe it or not. Written and mental reflections have allowed me to become a more appreciative person, which in turn has infused more positivity into my life.

Mental or written reflection is a cornerstone of many different belief systems around the world, and for good reason. Focusing on the positives makes the negatives seem to take up less space. This attitude change is an important step toward happiness. Counting your blessings fosters a sense of positivity and makes it a habit. This habit will help you stay happy even in times of stress, and allow you to derive joy from the little things.

FOCUSING ON WORK

The word "work" has a negative connotation for me. Whenever I think about "work," a feeling of dread swells inside of me as I think about completing necessary tasks. But just because a task is necessary doesn't mean it has to be tiresome. In fact, how can we be happy if we spend our days approaching our tasks with a bad attitude? Sure, work can be difficult and isn't necessarily always enjoyable, but there are benefits to work that can make you a more content person.

No matter what kind of work you do, there is always a sense of accomplishment that comes with completing it. Whether it's finishing a project for school or closing a deal with a company, there's a sense of satisfaction that comes with the conclusion of a nagging task. Even if I don't enjoy the process, I definitely enjoy the sense of fulfillment and encouragement that comes with completing an assignment. I feel capable knowing that I was able to accomplish this goal, and this capability translates into self-confidence, knowing that I can complete other goals. Finishing an essay makes me confident that I can finish not only other writings, but any challenges or tasks that school throws my way.

Work also provides an atmosphere of growth and challenge that we need. It stimulates our minds and constantly encourages us to push ourselves so that we can become better at what we do. Students can feel motivated to get better grades. Company workers can feel the drive to get a promotion. No matter what the environment, the mere act of being a part of it motivates you to excel at your chosen profession. Studies show that human beings need a sense of growth and motivation in order to be happy. We can't be happy when we are stagnant. We get happiness boosts whenever we grow and become more proficient. This explains the "big fish in a small pond" theory: most people feel happier and more confident when they are an expert in their chosen field, whether the expertise is being the most popular, the smartest, or the one with the most authority. Work provides us with an environment in which to excel.

In addition, work also supplies a challenge. In our early days of evolution, we had to forage for food for daily survival. Without the challenge of finding food, we wouldn't have had a sense of purpose—and we wouldn't have survived, for that matter. Although our challenges are no longer life-and-death scenarios, we still need them to keep us from becoming complacent. Who would be happy doing the same thing every single day without any change or challenge to shake things up? Without challenges we wouldn't be able to grow. Not only is the process of overcoming a challenge essential to our happiness, but the feeling of vanquishing that hurdle provides a rush of excitement and contentment. Next time you are confronted with a challenging task, try to look at it in a positive light instead of seeing it as a nagging task, and remind yourself that it will only make you a stronger person.

Work isn't always enjoyable, but it's necessary. Putting effort into your work may not bring immediate happiness, but the rewards of growing and changing in response to these tasks will help you feel happier and more self-confident. Seeing an A at the top of a paper I worked hard on fills me with more contentment and happiness than it would if I hadn't cared enough to try.

FAMILY

To say that we live busy lives is the understatement of the century. A plethora of responsibilities clamor for our attention as we try to fight off the sleep deprivation that constantly plagues us. It's difficult to find time for ourselves, let alone our families—so sometimes we neglect the very people that helped us grow into who we are today. I believe that we owe it to ourselves and our families to keep up with one another no matter what happens; after all, blood is thicker than water.

I advocate not just spending time with family, but spending *healthy* time with family. This means that there's no place for bickering, complaining, or contempt, as this will only cause tension and arguments. Focusing on the negativity in your relationships with family members will only push you further away from them.

According to psychotherapist Tracy Lamperti, spending time to foster a close-knit family creates a sense of trust that allows family members to rely on one another for support. Not only does this provide a sense of security, but this trust translates into a relationship where all parties can open up to and confide in one another. Personally, I can attest to this. I recently realized that I had grown distant from my parents and brother because I never carved time out of my schedule to dedicate to them. This became especially worrisome when I realized that I'm going to college in about a year, and I'll only see them once every few months. I decided I needed to make a change, and started off by spending more time with my younger brother. I didn't plan activities or anything, I just began to sit and talk to him while he was playing video games or watching TV in his room. Although at first I didn't really know what to say, the conversation would inevitably progress and soon he'd be telling me details about his personal life or experiences at school. Although this may not seem groundbreaking, it did create a sense of confidence and familiarity that translated to trust. We both slowly began to confide in each other and ask each other for advice; this provided both of us with not only a constant support system, but a trusted friend.

After reconnecting with my brother, I began to work on spending more time with my parents. After all, my parents had raised me and made numerous sacrifices for me, the least I could do was spend a little time with them. I began to accompany my mother on dog walks and sit with my father as he prepared a quick snack for himself. The simple act of talking to them created a sense of familiarity and trust. It's human nature to trust the people that you talk to all the time. Eventually, our mundane conversations progressed until I was asking my mom for advice concerning my personal life and talking to my dad about which colleges I want to apply to. And this new closeness benefited my parents too. I could see that they were happy to play an active role in their child's life and enjoyed talking to me, whether about serious subjects or more trivial stuff.

Lamperti also stresses that closer familial relationships can improve behavior. In young children, this can mean fewer temper tantrums, and in older individuals this can mean increased motivation and a better general attitude. I definitely think there is some validity to this. Personally, I watched my brother's grades increase as we became closer. This was not only because he felt comfortable asking me for help and advice about studying, but because we both motivated each other to work harder. I became more focused and organized as I became closer to my parents, and it wasn't because they were pushing me to excel any more than they normally do (this actually decreased, believe it or not). The closer I became to them, the more I was motivated to excel at whatever I was doing.

You may not experience the same benefits, but it's worth a shot. All "benefits" aside, becoming closer to my family really made me a happier person. I enjoyed spending time with my brother as we found more things that we had in common, and I genuinely liked being a support system in his life. The fact that we had developed a solid relationship comforted me and assured me that we would keep up with each other even when we were at college. I also genuinely enjoyed spending time with my parents. They were a lot more like me than I had initially thought (due to genetics, of course). I felt comfortable talking to them and found them to be a huge support system. They also began to trust me with more independence. It was a win-win situation.

So although we have busy schedules filled with friends and responsibilities, we shouldn't forget that at the end of the day family is also extremely important. Instead of taking them for granted, fostering a closer familial relationship can make us all happier.

SURROUNDING YOURSELF WITH POSITIVE PEOPLE

The people around you have a huge influence on your outlook, habits, and beliefs. Especially for young people, the company that we keep directly affects how we act and think on a daily basis. Surrounding yourself with negative people makes you think more negatively. Eventually, if you repeat this way of thinking long enough, it becomes a habit. The opposite is also true: when you surround yourself with positive people, you start to see the world more optimistically.

Most people think of negative people as "half glass empty" kind of people, but I'm also talking here about people who make you *feel* negatively—people who put you in a bad mood or somehow lower your self-esteem. While it's second nature to distance yourself from people who have a negative effect on your mood, sometimes it's hard to distance yourself from people who lower your self-esteem. I've seen and been in unhealthy friendships, and I've seen the effect they can have. Even if the person doesn't directly mean to put you down, sometimes their words can come off that way—even just off-the-cuff remarks can instantly dampen your mood. In fact, the person making these comments probably doesn't mean any harm by them the majority of the time, but nevertheless they can still be hurtful.

If you have a friend who fits this description, I suggest that you pull them aside and explain to them that their comments can be offensive. If the person doesn't change their habits after you've spoken with them, you may want to distance yourself from them. It can be difficult, but do you really want to spend your energy on a person that only sees and brings out the worst in you? Friends and colleagues should make you feel good about yourself and motivate you to do better, not belittle you.

People who constantly wallow in drama or gossip can also affect you negatively. While these people may be fun to hang around with, their negativity may eventually rub off on you. And if you think about it, people who say negative things about others will say negative things about you too.

It surprises me how many adolescents surround themselves with people that bring out the worst in them. This only exacerbates the prevalence of teenage depression, for it supplements the unhealthy thoughts that stem from this condition. Most of the time, we don't realize the consequences that these people have on us until after the fact.

ELIMINATING CLUTTER

Think about the last time you walked into your room and it was perfectly clean. How did that make you feel? Most of you probably felt calmer and more at ease. Even if you didn't, I dare you to tell me it had a negative effect on you. While it may seem tiresome to keep your room tidy, it's important to ensure that your surroundings are aesthetically pleasing. If you are happy with its appearance, you'll be happier there and more relaxed.

Clutter tends to exacerbate stress. A messy atmosphere fogs your mind. Clutter is also a constant reminder of impending chores, which can make you feel overloaded. By eliminating the clutter in your environment, you not only create an aesthetically pleasing atmosphere, but also eliminate some of the burdens in the back of your mind. Although there haven't been many studies about the effects of pleasing environments on happiness, the proof is in today's markets. Millions of dollars are spent each year on home improvement magazines, which praise organized environments. In addition, the success of stores such as The Container Store prove that there are millions of people who are at least hoping to become more organized. Personally,

I've found that having a clean room makes me feel more invigorated and relaxed.

Now that we've discussed the importance of a tidy space, now let's talk about how to get it. There are two main ways to eliminate clutter: get rid of things you don't need and put things back in their place. If we all search in the nooks and crannies of our rooms, we'll find objects that we haven't touched in years. While some of these items have sentimental value, others are only there because we haven't thrown them out sooner. While this may not seem like the most effective use of your time, I urge you to go through all drawers, table tops, etc. and throw out things that you don't use anymore, and won't in the future. It may be difficult to part with them if they have sentimental value, but I promise you really won't miss these items when they're gone.

Once you've completed this, half the battle is over. Unfortunately, the other half is harder to keep up with. Now that you have all of this newfound space, you need to organize your belongings—which I know is easier said than done. You may know where everything is supposed to go, but maybe laziness or other priorities have taken precedence over organizing your room. Now, however, I urge you to learn to take the extra two minutes to return your pajamas to your closet or to make your bed. It will have a tremendous effect on your space, and hence your mood. Clutter can be prevented if you take the time to return items to their proper place. By getting rid of old items and ensuring that clutter doesn't develop, you can transform a messy environment into a calming one.

Even though it may seem daunting to keep an organized environment, it won't get out of hand as long as you clear up a little each day. I assure you that the time you spend keeping your environment clean will pay off in the long run, when you have more peace of mind and feel happy in your surroundings.

SLEEP

Amongst everyday stresses and constant work we have one
source of bliss: sleep. Sleep is the only time when our brains
fully rest, even if only for a couple hours. It restores our bodies
and our minds, giving us energy to take on another day. But
although we all know the importance of sleep, few of us actually
get the amount of rest that we need. Sleep stays on the back
burner as daily responsibilities and stresses move to the
forefront of our minds. While I completely empathize with the
stress of responsibilities and a too-busy schedule, I urge you
reevaluate your time to ensure that you are getting enough sleep.

Most studies say that teenagers need around nine hours of sleep
per night. In a perfect world, we all would finish our work at a
reasonable hour and get to sleep on time. However, I know that
some days this is simply unrealistic. Instead, I urge you to aim
for around seven and a half hours of sleep during the week.
Although this is less than the recommended amount, it's still
more than a lot of people get. I know people who sleep four to
five hours a night, and trust me when I say that I see the
exhaustion on their faces. It might be difficult to carve this time

out of a busy schedule, but I promise you, it's completely worth it. The more time you spend asleep, the more alert you will be when you're awake—it's as simple as that. We can't expect our bodies to perform at their best unless we give them proper time to rest.

I also understand that hectic social lives sometimes don't allow for very much sleep on the weekends. See if you can set aside one day where you can sleep well. If you're going to a party on Friday night, try to get to sleep at a reasonable hour on Saturday night and sleep in Sunday morning. There should be at least one day during the week when you can get to sleep early, and one when you can let your body naturally wake up whenever it's ready to. Personally, I force myself to get to sleep at a reasonable time on Saturday nights (around 11) and don't set an alarm for Sunday morning. I usually wake up at around noon, feeling well rested and ready to tackle the load of homework that I have waiting for me.

Everyone knows the physical benefits of sleeping, but few know the mental benefits it provides. Studies have proven that sleep helps with overall happiness, because it regulates the amygdala. This part of the brain is responsible for controlling your emotions, and it becomes 60 percent more reactive when one receives a good night's sleep. A regulated amygdala prevents mood swings and allows your brain to effectively process and respond to emotions. In addition, sleep also combats stress by calming you down. It prevents you from becoming overly aggressive due to exhaustion and allows you to tackle obstacles with a clear head. It also heightens your critical thinking skills, memory, and concentration, qualities that are essential to performing well in a work or school environment. Overall, the mental benefits of sleep calm and stabilize you while increasing your overall happiness.

Since most of the physical benefits of sleep are well-known, I'm just going to explain a few of the less-known ones. First and foremost, sleep combats acne. Acne plagues millions of people every year and is one of the main causes of low self-esteem. A good night's rest regulates your body's glucocorticoid production, which in turn leads to better skin. In addition, sleep also strengthens your muscles and makes your workouts more effective. With a good night's rest, you'll be able to perform much better in any physical activity.

Sleep is a crucial part of our mental and physical health, and should be a priority. You'll feel rejuvenated after a restful night, and will be able to tackle the next day with more vigor.

EXERCISE

I get it, we all have extremely busy schedules with each minute in the day accounted for. You may be reading this title and thinking "How am I supposed to make time for one more activity, I barely have time to sleep." I completely understand these feelings and empathize with you, for I too have extremely busy days and short nights. But, I've come to realize that exercise is extremely important and should be a daily activity. Not only does science show us that it has a plethora of benefits, but I'm sure that you've experience this benefits each time that you've exercised. You can't possibly tell me that you feel worse after a good workout (unless you mean soreness).

The great thing about exercise is that it's effective even in small doses. Even if you can only squeeze in thirty minutes of exercise, I urge you to do so, for the results will be completely worth the tighter-packed schedule. If you really try to, I guarantee that you can find a small chunk of time for some daily exercise. If you have to get to school early, try exercising in the evening or at night, as a final step to a long day. If you can't find time at night, try exercising in the morning and let it invigorate and prepare you for the day ahead. No matter when you find the time to do so, exercise will be effective in boosting your mental and physical health.

Exercise has numerous physical benefits that can help you become a healthier person. It's the most effective way to burn calories, keep your internal organs healthy, and keep you fit. Some of these physical benefits will show up shortly after you begin to exercise, while others will be mostly internal. In addition to helping you become healthier, these physical benefits can also help you feel more confident about yourself. I think I speak for all of us when I say that we feel better about our appearance after a good workout. But, if the outwardly benefits aren't convincing enough, there are also numerous internal benefits that will help keep you healthy. Exercise has been known to regulate blood pressure, strengthen your bones and muscles, reduce your risk for many kinds of cancers, revitalize your heart, and increase your life expectancy. While many of you may feel that you don't directly need these benefits, I emphasize that even if you don't see the difference, your body becoming more capable and strong with every minute of exercise.

Everyone knows the physical benefits of exercise, but few know about the numerous mental and emotional ones. Although they are less known, these benefits are equivalent to the physical ones, if not better. The most common mental benefit is the release of endorphins, a chemical in your brain that is known to induce a positive feeling in the body. It also helps alleviate stress and serves as a healthy outlet for negativity. These benefits can improve your mood and help you feel happier on a daily basis. In addition, exercise is also known to curtail the effects of disorders such as ADHD, depression, and anxiety. If you don't suffer from these illnesses, exercise can help prevent them so that you won't have to deal with them in the future. In addition, the release of endorphins will make you feel happier and make your brain more alert. Not only will you feel the benefits of endorphins immediately, but you'll be happier in the long run with continued exercise.

We all know that exercise is extremely beneficial to the body, but science has proved that it's even more beneficial than most of us initially thought. It not only helps you feel more lively and happy, but it also keeps your internal organs running smoothly so you can lead a healthier lifestyle. Although it may be difficult to find time to include it in your daily routine, once it becomes a habit it'll become effortless. It's a simple task that can have life long effects, so I urge you to try to make some time for it.

THE OUTDOORS

Most of us spend the majority of our days either in a classroom or workplace. We spend hours upon hours hunched over dimly lit desks, often staring at a screen, as we rush to complete work before looming deadlines. With all of our stress and responsibilities, it can be difficult to find time for ourselves, let alone time to spend outside.

Studies show that our brains have evolved to detect slight changes in the environment and divert our focus whenever new stimulus reveals itself. This makes it extremely difficult for us to concentrate on a single task for a long period of time; our brains aren't made to work this way. Luckily, taking small breaks deactivates and then reactivates our brains so that we can focus more intensively on our work.

Spending some time outdoors maximizes your mental break. Studies have shown that spending time in nature can increase concentration. Frances Kuo and Andrea Taylor conducted a study that tested nature's impact on children who suffer from ADHD. Their data showed that children who spent more time outside showed fewer symptoms of ADHD than those who didn't. It helped them focus more effectively and gave them an energy boost. Spending time outdoors can also encourage you to be more active, which increases brain function. A brisk stroll in a park is an ideal way to revive your concentration so that you can finish your work more quickly and effectively. After all, what makes you feel more accomplished at the end of the day than knowing you've completed a nagging task?

Exposure to nature has also been known to reduce stress. Whether it's walking through a park or just sitting in your backyard, the natural setting has a knack for calming our minds. Studies show that exposure to nature reduces heart rate, clear proof that nature calms our bodies as well as our minds. In addition, the outdoors make us happier. Have you ever noticed that you feel more content after spending some time outside? Psychologists believe that our evolution causes us to have positive reactions to the safety associated with aspects of nature, such as a shady tree; elements that were previously helpful to our survival left imprints on our brains that allow us to feel safe and happy in their presence.

Not only does exposure to nature allow us to complete our responsibilities more efficiently, it also has positive effects on our brains and bodies that allow us to reduce stress and feel happier. If you can only squeeze the outdoors into your schedule by doing some work outside, great. These small benefits eventually add up to us becoming happier people.

YOU ARE WHAT YOU EAT

Have you considered the effect that your diet can have on your mood? What you eat can directly influence your attitude; the brain and stomach are more connected than you might expect. Consider adding a few foods into your diet (and deleting others), in order to feel more positive.

Fresh fruit provides a sensory experience that has been known to improve your mood. Take oranges, lemons, and other citrus fruits, for example. These citrus scents target neurotransmitters, to alleviate stress and act as a sort of immediate antidepressant. Studies show that citrus scents have a stimulating effect and make us feel more energized and happy. Another example of a stimulating scent is vanilla. It has a calming effect on the body and triggers a positive response in most people—not only because of positive associations we have with the scent, but because the scent itself provokes neurotransmitters to release chemicals to make you feel happier and more relaxed. Next time you're feeling stressed or overwhelmed, test out the calming effects of these scents.

Healthy foods are known to benefit physical and mental health. A study conducted by the Archives of General Psychiatry found that a Mediterranean diet had overwhelmingly positive effects on mental health. People who adhered to the diet—comprised of olive oil, vegetables, fish, and whole grains—reported 30 percent less depressive symptoms that those who didn't. The omega 3–rich oil in fish not only improves your physical health, but also causes your brain to release serotonin, which is known to regulate our mood.

Protein is also known to balance brain function and enhance mood, as well as regulate blood sugar levels, which prevents mood swings and irritability. Even eggs and nuts immediately stabilize glucose levels and prevent negative behavioral changes, proving that their benefits are not only physical, but also mental. Bananas are also another example of a mood-regulating food. In their simplest form, they contain dopamine, a chemical that directly alters your mood and makes you feel happier. They also contain B vitamins and magnesium, which soothe your nervous system and instantly make you feel more relaxed. The next one may come as a shock to some of you: coffee has a reputation among the scientific community for being an antidepressant. Coffee regulates many neurotransmitters in your brain that directly affect your happiness. It also heightens levels of BDNF (which provokes the creation of new neurons, making it essential to brain health), which has been known to combat symptoms of depression.

Just as there are many foods that increase happiness, there are also a plethora of foods that create mood swings and irritability. Take processed sugars, for example. Sugars actively lower

BDNF levels and cause inflammation in the body, which disrupts brain function and can cause depressive symptoms. While I admit that processed sugars are often the tastiest parts of some foods, they really aren't worth it when you examine the facts. Eating cake feels good in the moment, but its negative effects last much longer.

NEW YEAR'S RESOLUTIONS

I am notorious for abandoning my New Year's resolutions. Year after year I make them, but by the time February rolls around I've already given up on them. I used to see this as a negative, but recently I realized that maybe New Year's resolutions aren't that great. We make these resolutions at the start of every year, with the intention of trying to change ourselves. Some of these changes are healthy, but sometimes they move past healthy into the territory of impossible. Whether they fall on the side of healthy or impossible can be determined with these simple questions: Am I going against who I am? Am I making a change that could be unhealthy? If you answered "yes" to either of these questions, it's an impossible change, simple as that.

This is the main problem with New Year's resolutions: people set unrealistic or unhealthy goals, instead of accepting themselves for who they are. While it is certainly beneficial to set personal goals, self-acceptance is also important.

In some cases, New Year's resolutions are aimed at completely changing who you are. They can lead you to focus on your weaknesses instead of your strengths, which negatively impacts your opinion of yourself. Instead of trying to change weaknesses that cannot be changed, you might want to try accepting these qualities as a part of who you are. Self-improvement is crucial, but sometimes the most valuable thing you can do is improve your opinion of yourself, rather than thinking you have to change yourself.

The best way to have a more positive outlook on life is to begin with having a more positive outlook on yourself. Try to accept yourself for who you are—weaknesses and all. At the end of the day, the most important opinion that anyone can have of you is yours. Focusing on your strengths and accepting your weaknesses allows you to feel confident in yourself and to project an approachable aura. This positive outlook translates into your daily life, and makes focusing on the positives a habit.

New Year's resolutions can also undermine your past year's accomplishments. If you only focus on what's ahead, how can you fully appreciate what you've already achieved? For me, the most important part of a new year is reflecting on the old one, and realizing just how far you've come in a year's time. Even if it was not your best year, you did grow and become a better person and achieve something, no matter how small. While it is important to try to make the next year even better, it's also healthy for your self-esteem and positive mindset to acknowledge your achievements. Recognizing all the good moments of the past year will not only help you have a better year to come, but will have an indelible positive effect on your mind. Thinking positively is a habit, not something that just comes naturally. So, instead of feeling defeated about not accomplishing all of your New Year's resolutions, take some time to reflect on the great things you accomplished last year. At the end of the day, your opinion about yourself and the world around you is the most important factor that contributes to your overall happiness.

MENTAL BREAKS

Most of us have a constant list of responsibilities and obligations. Between school and work, there isn't much time left to relax and take care of yourself. Personally, I put my responsibilities first and myself second, which is effective but also leaves me exhausted. A couple of months ago, I had just taken the ACT, AP exams, and SAT subject tests and I was completely exhausted. I had spent every moment in the past month either studying or sleeping and hadn't left any time for myself, which left me feeling burnt out. I realized that I couldn't go on like this.

Sometimes there comes a time when you have to prioritize sanity over work. At one point, I needed to take a break and rejuvenate myself. I didn't put off my responsibilities, but I did start to find time in my busy schedule to do things that genuinely made me feel happy and relaxed. Even if it was for just half an hour, the mental break alleviated my stress, helped me feel less tired, and gave me a better attitude toward the work I had left. Even if it is a mundane activity such as watching TV, doing something you enjoy can not only distract you from your worries, it can also change your attitude and increase your positivity. This allows you to tackle each new responsibility with strength and energy, and brings more positivity to your daily life, which helps you to be happier in the long run.

There are many different ways to take a mental break and each of them has its merits. The most obvious one is sleeping, and while it may not be the most enjoyable activity, it will make you happier and more productive. Scientists recommend "power naps," which typically last from ten to thirty minutes and should take place before 4 PM. If the nap is any longer, you risk disrupting your sleeping schedule and waking up groggier than you were before you fell asleep. Personally, I feel rejuvenated and relaxed after a nap, which helps me attack my responsibilities with energy. Another kind of mental break is to do any activity that you really enjoy. This could be anything from watching an episode of *New Girl* (my favorite TV show) to reading your favorite book to going shopping with your friends. Doing something you enjoy will rejuvenate you and boost your positivity. A third kind of mental break is to do something physical. Spending hours at a desk can leave us feeling tired and sluggish, and more work will only exacerbate that. The best way to combat this lethargy and negativity is to be active. Personally, I like to go for a run—it gets my blood pumping and I get some contact with nature. The release of endorphins will also make you happier.

In addition to making your responsibilities more manageable, making time for yourself can also make you a happier person in general. If you can make some extra time for yourself, to do activities that genuinely make you feel more positive, you are that much closer to achieving happiness—which, in my opinion, is the main purpose of life.

MAKING NEW FRIENDS

The older we get, the less friends we seem to have. I guess it's just a fact of life that as people age, we make fewer friends and tend to hold on more tightly to the ones we already have. While this definitely isn't a bad thing, it's also not a particularly good thing either. As we mature, we tend to fear rejection more. Our qualities become more and more entrenched, and with that our image of ourselves takes shape. As that image becomes more and more developed, we tend to start fearing rejection of that image, which leads us to put ourselves out there less. While this is completely normal, we can often get stuck in this fear of rejection—until we stop putting ourselves out there completely.

You may be asking, what's wrong with that? There isn't anything wrong with this per se—we are just limiting ourselves and our opportunities. It's completely fine to have a small group of friends and cherish their friendship, but it can also be beneficial to open yourself up to new opportunities.

Making new friends can expose you to new experiences and new perspectives on life—new ideas and new perspectives that you normally wouldn't have any exposure to. This can be a great learning opportunity and can teach you valuable lessons about life, other people, and yourself. It's beneficial to get different people's opinions and ideas, because it helps you refine your own. I can't tell you how many times I've run a decision by someone who is very different from me and have benefitted greatly from it. The fresh perspective helps me see the situation in a different light, and often changes how I react to the situation.

New friends also bring new experiences and a variety of different adventures. Everyone has different ways of spending their time. Personally, my friends have encouraged me to try a variety of new experiences that I wouldn't have thought to try on my own. For example, my friend and I recently decided to explore Houston. We walked block after block and just went wherever we felt like going for the entire day. Throughout the course of the day, we tried tons of new food, explored the underground tunnels, and saw some cool art in a museum. Though it doesn't seem like much, this experience was amazing and I know I'll remember it for years to come. In addition, I learned more about myself: that I truly love cities and I love exploration. I wouldn't have known this about myself if my friend and I hadn't spent the day together.

New friends also give us a sense of companionship, which is essential to all people. We thrive in environments where we are supported and cared for, around friends and loved ones. Making new friends offers us more opportunities to find the people who may end up supporting us and giving us the sense of camaraderie that we need in our daily lives. This shared sense of companionship can make both parties happier on a daily basis. You may think that you already have plenty of friends who love and support you, but one can never really have too many friends. More friends provide more companionship and more happy times, it's as simple as that.

In life, we rarely seek out new opportunities for happiness— most of the time they arise on their own and leave us wondering how we ever lived without them. Although you may not be actively seeking a new friend, one might come into your life, and later you may question how you lived without them. Life brings unexpected gifts, but only if you're open to them. Sometimes, actively seeking new opportunities is the best way to open yourself up to them.

COMPARING YOURSELF TO OTHERS

One of the most detrimental blows to our self-confidence is comparing ourselves to others. It's a natural impulse that feeds off our need for gratification and becomes reinforced when we perform better than others. This can make us feel more capable and can elevate us in our mental hierarchy. However, while this impulse can sometimes give us a temporary self-esteem boost, it can also do more damage than good. When we don't measure up to our peers, it can make us feel inadequate, which is injurious to our motivation and self-esteem. This can hurt our self-image and keep us from being the best that we can be. I'm sure every one of us has suffered the belittling results of comparing ourselves to others.

When you compare yourself to someone else, you are essentially looking at yourself according to their standards, which are completely different than yours. Since we are often comparing our weaknesses to other people's strengths, this process can leave us feeling bad about ourselves. Believing that you aren't as worthy as someone else can destroy your self-image, creating a negativity that prevents you from being content with yourself. This keeps you from being the best that you can be and can diminish your motivation.

One of the fundamental flaws in comparing yourself to others is the fact that each and every one of us is totally different. We have distinct, unique strengths and weaknesses. Comparing yourself to others is like comparing apples and oranges. For example, you might be an incredible athlete who isn't book-smart. If you compare yourself to someone who makes straight A's, you're going to feel bad about yourself. We can't all fit the same mold, so it's pointless to compare everyone using the same criteria.

In addition, the very process of comparing yourself to others is flawed. Measuring yourself to other people's standards won't have any effect on your abilities. You will not be more or less skilled after the process; you'll just have a different opinion of yourself, usually a less positive one. Either you'll overestimate or underestimate your abilities—either way, they won't really change. Your opinion of yourself will change, but you won't really change at all. The energy you spent is totally wasted, because it doesn't actually yield beneficial results. At the end of the day, you can only be the best version of yourself, so it's pointless to compare yourself to the best version of someone else.

We humans seem to have an innate need to compare ourselves to others. More often than not, this leaves us feeling bad about ourselves, which is poisonous to any sort of motivation. Instead, I believe it's infinitely more important to focus this attention on self-improvement, so that you can be the best and happiest version of yourself.

OUR APPEARANCES

Some people believe that focusing on your appearance fosters the superficiality that currently plagues our society. I think this is an oversimplification of the problem. Yes, people shouldn't get too caught up in their appearance, but there is nothing wrong with taking pride in how you look. Feeling good about how you look can give you a self-confidence boost that allows you to carry yourself with ease, have a healthier mental attitude, and be a more positive, happy person.

Improving your appearance means something different to everyone. We can all probably think of five small things that we can do to make ourselves happier with our appearance on a daily basis. One of those things for me was working on clearing my skin. My skin was the bane of my existence until I finally decided to do something about it. Since nothing else was working, I decided to go to the dermatologist, and thankfully the creams she prescribed worked like a charm. Looking back, I'm so thankful that my dermatologist was able to help, because my self-image has never been better. I've also taken other small measures to improve my appearance on a daily basis. I spend five to ten minutes to do my makeup and hair each morning, which helps me feel better about myself throughout the day. It's a small effort, but feeling put together just puts me in a better mood and helps me feel confident. Sometimes small, quick efforts can make a big difference in our day.

While small measures are effective in improving self-confidence, some of us are looking for larger-scale solutions. Please consider whether what you're considering is healthy. Nothing is worth potentially harming yourself, either physically or mentally, so I urge you to consider the risk factor in anything that you pursue. If there's little risk involved, I urge you to go for it with everything you've got. Personally, last summer I decided that I wanted to become more fit. I was a skinny girl who didn't have much muscle, and I wanted to be more toned. I wasn't unhappy with my body at all, but I felt that becoming more fit would help me feel happier and healthier, so I decided to pursue it. I began to go to the gym almost every single day, and in a few short weeks I began to see results. My arms and legs became toned, and I felt way better about myself as a result. This was a big change in lifestyle, but it made me a healthier person.

Many people believe that focusing on your appearance is detrimental to your self-image, but I disagree. Your appearance is one of the most important expressions of yourself, so it's only natural to connect your appearance to your self-esteem. While your appearance definitely shouldn't be the sole factor determining your self-confidence, it can positively affect your self-image if you let it. Making small physical or lifestyle changes can help you feel better about yourself in ways that internal changes can't.

PLANNING YOUR LIFE

From the minute we enter elementary school, people begin to ask, "What do you want to be when you grow up?" Most of us had a pretty clear idea of who we wanted to be at that time. However, it doesn't stay this easy. As the years go by and we change, so does our vision of the future. The idea of ourselves that fit so perfectly with who we wanted to be doesn't fit so perfectly anymore. We may not really know what we want to pursue anymore. And that's okay.

Some people may have their whole future planned out, but most of us don't, and there's nothing wrong with that. We're just beginning our journeys, so it's fine if we don't know exactly where we're going. People may tell you that youth is meant for making the decisions that will create the pathway to the rest of your life. While I do believe that this is true, I also think it's an exaggeration. As young people, we should experiment and try new things until we find our "passion," but these passions aren't as indelible as people make them out to be. We may entertain a plethora of interests before finding one that sticks, and that's okay. There's no rush to grow up. In fact, the longer we take to make these important decisions, the better the chance we'll make the right one. The more possibilities we consider, the more likely we'll choose one (or more!) that's right for us.

We can't allow ourselves to become stressed out at the thought of the future. Every day I see people around me spending more time thinking about the future than they do about the present. They waste the present on thoughts of the future. They think they should have everything figured out, but the fact of the matter is that there is a time and a place for everything. If we obsess about the future, get caught up in thoughts of college and professions, we let the everyday moments slip by. In order to be happy, it's helpful to lower the amount of stress in your life and appreciate your life right now.

I think if you have faith in yourself, eventually everything will work out for the best. You may make some mistakes. Even those who have their entire lives planned out make mistakes and encounter obstacles (and change their minds)—and you will too, but these mistakes will make you stronger and more capable of handling future situations.

THE ARGUMENT AGAINST GOSSIPING

Gossiping is a part of human nature—we all do it at some time or another. While it might be fun in the moment, gossiping can bring unnecessary negativity into your life. It can also distract you from focusing on your own happiness, since you're so caught up in thinking negatively about other people's lives. It has a snowball effect: you say one benign comment about someone and then the person you're talking to follows up with a slightly worse one. You retort with an even harsher comment, until you both are belittling the third party. It may seem harmless, but these comments often get back to the person they're about, and when they do they may sting a lot more than you intended.

Personally, I feel very guilty after gossiping about someone. Even if you don't feel guilty, gossiping puts you in a pessimistic state of mind. We all know that gossiping brings negativity into many people's lives, negativity that can plague other people for years to come. It also damages people's opinion of you, which in turn will make you feel bad about yourself. Even worse, knowing that you made someone else unhappy will lower your own opinion of yourself.

So, consider the consequences before saying something that you may regret. There's enough negativity in the world without us adding to it.

MONEY

Money is a sensitive topic. Some people see it as a mark of power and others see it as a means to make life more comfortable. Either way, most people are conflicted as to whether money itself can be a source of happiness. While I definitely don't think money is the key to happiness, I believe that it can be a source of happiness as long as you keep it in perspective. Sometimes people think being rich will solve all of their problems, but in reality this just isn't true. It may eliminate a few problems, though, and it can definitely improve aspects of your life.

Studies show that richer people tend to be happier. According to a study conducted by the Pew Research Center, families with a higher income tend to characterize themselves as happy more often than families with a lower income. But I think there's more to this situation than meets the eye. I think it's not the presence of money, but rather the *lack* of money that affects happiness. It seems reasonable to assume that families who feel stress about making ends meet would be less happy than families who don't have this worry. It isn't necessarily that the presence of money makes you feel happy, but that the lack of having to worry about it can make you more content. In addition, the alleviation of this material stress allows people to focus on other goals, which could be a big source of happiness.

Happiness comes from a feeling of self-satisfaction, security, and connection with others. While money doesn't guarantee these feelings, the way you use money can greatly affect how you feel about yourself, your situation, and others. Personally, I use money to improve my daily life. If I am struggling with a particularly difficult situation and money could alleviate some of the stress associated with it, then I feel completely justified in spending the extra dollars to make my life easier. For example, when I first started writing these essays I was typing and researching on a sluggish computer that distracted me from writing and prolonged the process. I quickly realized that struggling with my computer not only irritated me, but made me dread writing, which should have been a source of joy. It was then that I made the decision to use my savings to buy myself a new computer, a decision that I have never regretted. Sure, it may have cost a lot of money and probably wasn't completely necessary, but it allowed me to derive joy from something important to me on a daily basis, and that, in my opinion, is priceless.

There are plenty of other instances in which money has made me feel more content, but there is another that particularly sticks out in my memory. I clearly recall walking the isles of Nordstroms with my best friend when I stumbled upon a pair of pants at the TopShop counter. Believe me when I tell you that these pants were perfect. The waist fit snugly but wasn't suffocating. The material was soft and lay smoothly on my skin without being too clingy. The mid-rise, skinny cut was uber flattering for my legs and waist. In short, these pants made me feel a million times better about myself. While not all of you will understand these pant's perfection, I hope that you can resonate with the idea that they were an instant confidence-booster. I knew I had to buy them until I realized that I had already spent way too much on clothes in the past month. However, I realized that these pants truly made me feel happy, and what was the point of spending money if it wasn't to make me feel happier? Sure, these pants weren't a necessity and prevented me from shopping for a while, but every time I put on those pants I feel content and don't regret my decision. The key to these two purchases is that they both continuously make me feel happy, they weren't just an impulse buy that made me feel happy for a day. Purchases, however large or small, are only worthwhile to your happiness if they provide more than just instant gratification.

However, I am by no means advocating spending money needlessly. If you genuinely can't afford a purchase, for example, it would probably be detrimental to your happiness rather than beneficial. The key to spending money wisely is to spend it cautiously and thoughtfully, on items that you genuinely think will improve your daily routine—even something as simple as a new candle that would improve your experience while doing homework.

The effect of money on happiness is an enigma that differs for every person. Some value it as a means to a comfortable life, and some see it as a mark of their personal success. Whether or not you agree, I think we can all agree that money can supplement happiness. Personally, I am fortunate enough to not have to worry about making enough money to sustain my lifestyle, which allows me to use money to help me feel more content on a daily basis. While money does not buy happiness, careful spending can help you feel more satisfied, secure, and connected with others.

FRIENDS

I know, this one seems like a no-brainer. But people tend to forget this. With our busy lives, we can forget to foster the very relationships that make us happy. We all know that friends are important, but how many of us consistently carve out time to spend with them or work on fostering a closer relationship with them? The first step in becoming closer to your friends is spending time with them, not on social media but in person.

Epicurus once said, "Of all the things that wisdom provides for living one's entire life in happiness, the greatest by far is the possession of friendship." I could not agree more. The need for companionship is ingrained in each and every one of us, and if satisfied, that need can provide an abundance of happiness. Studies show that people tend to be happier when surrounded with people, no matter what activity they're doing. Personally, I realized that I was inconsistent and unhappy working out alone. I had a gym schedule, but I would often skip a day and watch TV instead. I came to the realization that working out would probably be more enjoyable if I had a workout buddy, so I called up one of my friends and we decided to go to the gym together every day. This plan was extremely successful. Not only did we only skip one day over the course of a month, but we also became closer friends, which made me happy. Not only does friendship make you happier, but scientists have shown that it increases lifespan, reduces your risk of depression, boosts immunity, and encourages you to avoid unhealthy habits.

But how do you become closer to your friends? It's simple: start with spending more time with them. Instead of hanging out at home alone, call up a friend and go out to eat with them, or have them come over to make dinner together. Most of my closest friends became my closest friends because of the amount of time that we spent together. My best friend and I came to be best friends because of a school trip. We were assigned to the same hotel room by chance, and we were both unhappy about it. I clearly remember thinking, "I barely know this girl, this is going to be so awkward." Well, it wasn't. After two hours of being forced into each other's company, we were hysterically laughing and binging on Cheez-Its. Sometimes all it takes is some bonding for two people to become closer.

The next step to becoming closer to your friends is to be a good friend. Aristotle says that the closest form of friendship is based on virtue, meaning that both friends wish the best for each other and help each other attain their best. It seems simple, but it entails not only generosity but at times selflessness. Being a good friend takes practice and patience, as it's hard to not always put yourself first. But not only do I feel happiness when I act virtuously, my friends notice it too; they feel closer to me and are more inclined to act virtuously toward me. In fact, a turning point in one of my friendships was based on virtue. A friend called me crying the night before a final because she had just gone through a breakup. Although I had tons of studying to do, I spent an hour consoling her and telling her that she would eventually move on. The next day, she sent me a long text thanking me for being such a good friend. I could genuinely feel her appreciation. Weeks later, when I was feeling stressed, I called her and she consoled me for hours. Friendship is a two-way street, but sometimes we have to take the first step.

I've been talking about developing new friendships a lot, but we can't disregard old friends. Old friends have seen us in our awkward stages and loved us even when we weren't so lovable. I understand that old friends can drift apart, but sometimes it's worth bringing them back into our lives even if just in a small way. For example, I reconnected with my childhood best friend a couple months ago. We got back in touch when she followed me on Instagram. When I saw her name pop up on my phone, memories came flooding back of countless sleepovers and made-up games. I sent her a quick message asking how she was and soon we began to talk about old times. She hasn't become one of my best friends again, but it was nice to think about old memories. Talking to her brought back the past for a couple of hours and it genuinely made me happy. No matter how far you've come, old, happy memories can always make you smile.

I can personally attest to the fact that close friendships make you happier. Over the course of the past two years, I've made new friends and fostered closer friendships that I think will accompany me throughout life. The fact that I've deeply bonded with these friends makes me enjoy their company all the more. I feel as if I can talk to them about pretty much anything and they are a huge support system in my life. We've become so close that we have fun while doing absolutely nothing, and I am extremely grateful for that. The pure, simple happiness that I derive from spending time with my best friends is matched by few other things. My friends and I love each other, and we are the happiest when we're spending time together.

THE PAST

The past is all we know, and it makes up the majority of our perception of life. Good or bad, it has shaped us into the people that we are today. Every single experience has taught us a lesson, whether it be about pain or happiness. Although the past is the only part of life that is completely certain, at the end of the day it has passed. It's completely gone, completely unalterable. Many people spend their life thinking about the past or fixating on it. This is useless, simply because we are all completely different people than we were in the past. We have grown with every passing day. As hard as it may sometimes be, it's more beneficial to look at the present with fresh eyes. Yes, it is important to learn from the past, but you can't let that knowledge taint your present or your future; instead you should use it as a guide while still keeping an open mind.

I lived my early high school life in the past. I couldn't live up to my true potential because I was constantly fixating on my past limitations. Every time I wanted to do something new or something that took even an ounce of courage, my mind would drift to thoughts of my past failures and I would stop in my tracks. I wouldn't allow myself to become the person I wanted to be because I kept fixating on people's past perceptions of me. I had grown to become an extroverted person, but it was difficult for me to show that aspect of myself because I knew that everyone still thought of me and treated me like a quiet, shy kid. I constantly held myself back because of my fear of people's reaction to my change. I was letting my past self and my classmates' past selves stop me from growing and changing. It seems absurd, but the past will make you do absurd things sometimes! Thankfully, I eventually grew out of my fearful stage and embraced the person I had become. At first, people were shocked, because it was almost as if I'd done a 180—but they got used to it. Even the kid who used to tease me for my shyness noticed my change and befriended me. The results were completely different than I had expected. The only thing holding me back was my past perception of myself—nobody else cared.

Often, past failures hinder people from moving forward. I have watched people in my life fixate on past events or past misfortunes until it mentally cripples them. They never let go of the disappointment and pain, and it constantly throbs in the back of their minds. This kind of thinking is not only toxic, but it keeps you from learning from the past. Instead of learning from your failures, this way of thinking sets you up for another failure. Mistakes can be difficult, but at the end of the day they aren't truly mistakes if you learn from them, they're simply learning experiences.

I watched a friend of mine wistfully remember a past relationship for months. The relationship had ended because her boyfriend thought that she was too "demanding" and that she would burden him with her stress. One day he decided that it wasn't a healthy relationship for him and told her that they should break up. However, she wasn't ready to let go and constantly pushed him to take her back, promising that she would change. Her insistence that they should get back together only further alienated him. In the coming weeks, I tried to comfort my friend and explain to her that she would eventually meet someone new, but to no avail. Love is hard and sometimes it's difficult to move on, but at the end of the day we can't keep knocking on a closed door. My devastated friend kept doing just that. Even months later, she regretted her actions and wished that she and her ex-boyfriend could resume their relationship, but he had already moved on. Eventually, after long talks with close friends, she realized that the relationship was over and that all she could do was change her future actions. She realized that although the end of the relationship wasn't entirely her fault, she could have been less "demanding" and "burdensome." Her experience was painful, but it taught her a valuable lesson for the future.

I know forgetting the past is easier said than done. But the past has slipped from our fingertips, so we can't let our memories of it haunt us. We have to focus on the present and prepare for the future to truly be happy. We can't erase a sad past, but we can use it to create a happy future. Every event can be a learning experience if you make it one. It's easier to live without regrets if you know that the lessons that you've learned from the past are preparing you for a happier future. It's hard to let go, but sometimes we have to in order to live a fulfilling and happy future.

MUSIC

This essay is probably a lot more personal than the rest and may not resonate with everyone, but that's okay. Music is known to provide happiness and enjoyment, but I'm not sure if it provides the same kind of happiness for everyone. Personally, I adore music, and not just in the "I listen to music when I'm bored" kind of way. Music can make me feel any emotion at any time, and I know that it can have this effect on others too. I've always been drawn to it and have realized that it helps me cope in almost any uncomfortable situation.

I clearly remember a day in the life of my nine-year-old self, when my parents got into a heated argument. I listened to them argue for hours behind the closed door of my room. I was convinced that they would get a divorce and cried throughout their argument. Just when I felt like I would explode from all the emotion, my cousin walked into the room and sat on the bed with me. She explained that my parents probably wouldn't get a divorce, but that I should have a good cry anyway to get all of my emotions out. She played "Breakeven" by the Script on repeat and I cried for a solid ten minutes. Surprisingly, it made me feel a whole lot better; afterward, I felt like I would be able to cope with it even if they did get a divorce. Looking back, I laugh every time I think of this story, but the fact is that the sappy song helped me in my time of need. It gave me confidence and made me feel as if someone was empathizing with me, even if it was just the voice of a stranger.

Music can also transport you to a completely different time; think of it as a mental time machine. According to a recent study by Jeremy Hsu, the prefrontal cortex creates and stores an association between music and particular memories. Although I (and many others who experience this) had a sneaking suspicion that this was true, science's validation proves to me that music plays an important role in our lives. Anyway, it's not particularly important how this phenomenon happens, just that it does. I can't tell you how many times music has brought me back to a happy memory and completely made my day. Just a few days ago, my friend and I were driving to the mall when an old favorite came on the radio. We both immediately looked at each other and remembered a moment two summers ago when we were listening to this song in the car. It was a beautiful day and a bunch of us were driving to a graduation party while belting this song at the top of our lungs. It was the beginning of summer so we were particularly happy that day, and the song's catchy chorus was the perfect tune for a bunch of teenage girls to sing in the car. The song only lasted three minutes, but hearing it again brought us both back to that exact moment and made me happier for the rest of the day.

I've also found that good music has a knack for making any situation more enjoyable. Whenever there's a good song playing in the background I have infinitely more fun. There's just something about dancing and singing to a great song that makes you forget every worry in the world, even if it is just for a few minutes. I actually just experienced this yesterday, which is what prompted me to write this essay. A friend and I were in the car driving to a restaurant when she played one of our favorite songs. We both immediately started singing and dancing until we were laughing hysterically while still trying to yell the words to the song. After it was over, she remembered a funny story and recounted it as we both laughed for the rest of the car ride. It seems simple, but it was one of those blissful moments when you forget every little worry and just feel the euphoria swelling inside of you. My friend had just gone through a painful breakup, but she told me she didn't think about it for that car ride and forgot the pain she was going through. It's as if music engulfed both of our minds in glee, and made us forget about everything else. I can't explain why, but the happiness I felt in that moment was matched by few things and I'll remember it for a long time.

It's crazy to think that a simple song could have such an impact on us, yet it does. Music has a knack for making your worries disappear for a few minutes. Some of my funniest memories involve music and some of my happiest moments have a song playing in the background. Personally, I don't care whether it's the prefrontal cortex or the beat of the song that provides this exhilaration, all I know is that music makes me indubitably happy.

HIGH SCHOOL

I've noticed that with each passing generation, teenagers seem to become more and more focused on high school. In our parents' time, students led full lives outside of the school environment, but nowadays school is the center of every student's life, whether it be academically or socially or both. Kids no longer learn outside of the school environment, and focus most of their attentions on climbing the social ladder within their given school. While it is only natural that we focus on excelling at the place where we spend the most of our time, I've noticed that this can consume many. It seems like a this lack of outside stimulation and reevaluation of students' priorities has had some devastating effects on our generation as a whole that will only get worse as with time.

Excelling academically at school is important. It is the baseline of the college admissions process and can lead the way to a strong career. Good grades are something that every student should strive for and prioritize. However, there is a huge difference between getting good grades and *learning*.

Personally, I can get A's without learning much at all. I memorize and understand information for an assessment, but don't truly learn it that well. I end up forgetting it a couple of days after the assessment, because learning isn't my priority, grades are. Although most of us spend our formative years like this, I don't think it's a healthy approach. Memorization doesn't satisfy the innate curiosity that each and every one of us has; in fact, it eliminates it.

I used to be an insanely curious child. I began researching and blogging at the ripe old age of 12. I was an avid reader who read everything from nonfiction to classics and I kept up with the latest news about technology so I could blog about it. But as school became more time consuming and achieving good grades became more of a wearisome task, the time for my extra learning activities ended. I stopped blogging, because I didn't really have time for it, and I started to sleep instead of read. These activities weren't interesting to me anymore. I was getting top grades, but I wasn't satisfying my curiosity; in fact, I had eliminated it. I was also significantly more stressed and less happy than I was when I was learning for myself; the joy I'd gotten from learning about topics that interested me was gone.

Finally, I realized that I needed to go beyond grades and get back to being curious. I craved that feeling of wanting to know more about something for personal growth. I started to take time out of my schedule to really reflect on myself and find out what it was that I was actually interested in. I read random articles and tried to expose myself to new topics until I found something that sparked some sort of interest, and eventually I learned that I am interested in psychology. Now, even if my schedule is jam-packed, I find half an hour to read a book about behaviorism or to write part of an essay. This not only renews my innate curiosity and makes me happier, but I believe that it makes me genuinely smarter and more well-read. There's a difference between being intelligent and getting good grades, and that difference begins with curiosity.

For many, high school is a place of not only academic achievement, but also social achievement. It's one thing to be at the top of your class and another thing to be *at the top* of your class. If you're in high school, you know what I'm talking about. Most high school students are obsessed with being popular. As cliché as this sounds, it's completely true—at least at my school. High-schoolers want to have as many friends as possible and want to be friends with (or be) the kids that get invited to everything. It's human nature and it's unavoidable, but at the end of the day we need to realize that there is life outside of this environment; the world is bigger than high school. There are billions of people who don't go to your school and these people are all waiting for you in the real world. Most of them don't care how many parties you were invited to in high school.

Popularity is temporary and soon we will all be placed in a completely new environment where this process will start back up again. Everything you worked for high school will be gone, and you'll be left with a clean slate. This is why it's important to have goals and true friends outside of your high school social life. The memories that you make with these friends will last forever; the goals that you fulfill will stay with you throughout your life.

I know what it's like to get caught up in the high school social scene. In fact, I take pride in my social standing and like being friends with the majority of my school; I don't deny myself popularity just because it's temporary. I'm still a cheerleader and hang out with the popular girls in my grade because I genuinely like them. However, I've also worked to create a fulfilling life outside of that popularity. Some of my best friends don't even go to my school, and when I'm with them my social standing doesn't matter. We eat out, laugh, and make memories that have nothing to do with school, and these are memories that I'll remember forever. I know that I'll be friends with them long after high school and it make me happy to know that I'll have them even when high school fades from our memories.

I'm not saying that your social standing in high school shouldn't matter, just that it isn't the *only* thing that matters. If you focus on having genuine friends and making memories that won't fade, and you're popular in the process, great. I've also made sure that I keep myself busy with outside goals and projects so that I don't forget the true purpose of life. High school isn't the center of my world. The center of my world is what I accomplish in life and the kind of person I am, which is why most of my efforts and attention are focused on that. I'll admit, I used to get caught up with high school drama, but now I make a concerted effort to make and fulfill personal goals that have nothing to do with school. High school's ephemeral nature makes it impossible for it to be the center of my life, and so I make sure that my life is also peppered with indelible memories and goals.

High school is an important part of a student's life, but at the end of the day we only have four years in high school's little bubble before we are propelled into the real world, and we need to make sure that we are ready for it when it comes. Grades and popularity should never take the place of curiosity, goals, and true friends. These are the things that make life truly fulfilling. We should focus on excelling in life in general—in high school and in other avenues. It's a big world out there, and we only stifle our potential if we focus all of our attention on excelling in a temporary environment.

BEING SINGLE AND FINDING YOURSELF

It seems like "love" is constantly around us, whether in movies like *Sleepless in Seattle,* or Instagram "couple goals." It's hard to escape the constant chatter of people admiring cute couples or wishing that they were part of one. True, relationships are a natural part of life, but the very idea of them can become all-consuming. Social media isn't helping by providing the perfect platform for showcasing seemingly perfect relationships. But the truth is, no relationship is perfect.

It's almost as if being single has become some sort of curse. People, especially adolescents, long to be in a relationship and to be part of all the cuteness that goes along with it. Things in life come and go, and relationships are just the same. They'll eventually come, and they don't need to be a source of anxiety in the meantime. Girls and boys around the world are putting themselves under a microscope to figure out why they are single and how they can change that fact ASAP. It's an unnecessary stress that keeps people from being content in their lives as they are.

Many people measure their self-worth at least partially by whether or not they have a significant other. Not only is this unhealthy, it puts your self-confidence in a constant state of fluctuation. If you're relying on someone else for your own self-worth, it's impossible to have a sturdy sense of self-confidence. I understand that relationships can provide an ego boost, but at the end of the day this other person's opinion of you is not more important than yours.

So, for those of you that aren't in a relationship, don't worry about it. There isn't any rush to attach yourself to someone else; we all have plenty of time ahead of us to be in plenty of different relationships. In the meantime, focus on yourself and make time for self-improvement. When you do get into a relationship, you'll have much less time for yourself—and your friends—so it's good to use the time while you have it.

People seem to have a misconception about being single—they think it means you're lonely or sad, or there's something wrong with you. But most single people are just ordinary people living their daily lives. They might feel sad or lonely sometimes, but ultimately they're content with themselves and their friends. And that's how I think it should be. Don't stress yourself out trying to find a significant other—it'll eventually happen, I promise. Instead, use your energy to become the best possible version of yourself, so that when your person comes into your life you're ready.

Works Cited

"Friendships: Enrich Your Life and Improve Your Health." *Mayo Clinic*,
    Mayo Foundation for Medical Education and Research, 5 Feb.
    2014, www.mayoclinic.org/healthy-lifestyle/adult-health/in-
    depth/friendships/art-20044860.

Hsu, Jeremy. "Music-Memory Connection Found in Brain." *Live
    Science*, Purch, 24 Feb. 2009, www.livescience.com/5327-
    music-memory-connection-brain.html.

Kuo, Frances E., and Andrea Faber Taylor. "A Potential Natural
    Treatment for Attention-Deficit/Hyperactivity Disorder:
    Evidence from a National Study." *U.S. National Library of
    Medicine*, National Center for Biotechnology Information, U.S.
    National Library of Medicine, Sept. 2004, A Potential Natural
    Treatment for Attention-Deficit/Hyperactivity Disorder:
    Evidence From a National Study.

Lamperti, Traci. "The Benefits of Family Time." *Traci Lamperti*,
    www.tracylamperti.com/pdfs/3Family%20Time.pdf.

"Parallels between the Science of Happiness and the Philosophy of
    Friendship." *The Pursuit of Happiness*, Pursuit of Happiness,
    www.pursuit-of-happiness.org/science-of-
    happiness/communicating/links-to-the-philosophy-of-happiness/.

"Real Charity." *BuddhaSasana*,
    www.budsas.org/ebud/whatbudbeliev/168.htm.

Rubin, Gretchen. *The Happiness Project: Or, Why I Spent a Year Trying
    to Sing in the Morning, Clean My Closets, Fight Right, Read
    Aristotle, and Generally Have More Fun*. Harper Collins
    Publishing, 2011.

---. "'The Pure Act of Working towards Something and Accomplishing It

Makes Me Happier.'" *Gretchen Rubin*, 3 Jan. 2013,
gretchenrubin.com/happiness_project/2013/01/the-pure-act-of-
working-towards-something-and-accomplishing-it-makes-me-
happier/.

Schwartz, Tony. "Why Appreciation Matters so Much." *Harvard
Business Review*, Harvard Business School Publishing, 23 Jan.
2012, hbr.org/2012/01/why-appreciation-matters-so-mu.html.

Seiter, Courtney. "The Science of Taking Breaks at Work: How to Be
More Productive by Changing the Way You Think about
Downtime." *Buffer Open*, 21 Aug. 2014,
open.buffer.com/science-taking-breaks-at-work/.

Wise, Abigail. "Here's Proof Going Outside Makes You Healthier."
Huffington Post, 22 June 2014,
www.huffingtonpost.com/2014/06/22/how-the-outdoors-make-
you_n_5508964.html.

ABOUT THE AUTHOR

Ayelah Iqbal is a high school senior living in Houston, Texas. Her previous works include the blogs: appleinquirer.com, techforteenagers.com, and studentbehaviorst.com.

www.ingramcontent.com/pod-product-compliance
Lightning Source LLC
Chambersburg PA
CBHW050502290526
45786CB00006B/2393